DECIPHERING THE ADDICTED BRAIN

A Guide to Understanding and Helping a Loved One Towards Recovery

CORNEL N. STANCIU, M.D., M.R.O.

To my wife who has always supported my endeavors

and motivated me to pursue my dreams ---

TABLE OF CONTENTS

ACKNOWLEDGEMENTS

I would like to thank my wife Samantha, my parents Cornel and Liliana and my grandparents Ionel and Consuela who have constantly provided me with support, taught me that nothing is impossible, and encouraged me to always pursue my passions regardless of how impossible they may seem. I would also like to thank my mother and father-in-law Karla and Karunan for all their encouragement and support.

I would not be in the position I am today, let alone have the opportunity to share my expertise through this book, if it were not for the wonderful mentors I have had throughout my career that supported my growth as a physician. Particularly, I would like to acknowledge Dr. Thomas Penders' influence in my career path and for guiding me to a position of leadership in the field of Addictions.

At the foundation of everything I do on a daily basis stand the patients whom I have cared for and who have taught me what it is like to suffer from an addiction disorder and how my treatment can restore their lives.

*Editing and peer review for this book provided by Nikhil Teja, MD

PREFACE

I have treated multiple individuals throughout my career and to uphold my ethical obligations, I have relied on a variety of strategies to protect their identities and privacy throughout this book while concurrently providing relevant examples to the readers. The patients in this book do not represent any real persons. Any resemblance to a particular person is accidental, inadvertent, and unintended. Despite the aforementioned, I have no doubt that some might read this book and say, "this is me". I regard this as evidence that I have provided an accurate representation of the experience of our patients.

I would like to point out that throughout this book you will come across the term "substances". By this I am referring to all drugs and alcohol products that have addictive potential.

WHY I TREAT ADDICTION

Often I am approached by fellow physicians, other colleagues, patients and their families with the question of why I chose my current specialty. Do I have no other choice? Is it financially rewarding? Do I have an addiction myself? Do I just enjoy the pain of dealing with a highly stigmatized, high profile, disease? As physicians, especially when certain treatment outcomes end in disappointments or defeats, I think it is very important to step back and reflect on the work we do and define a "mission statement" simply put, the reason why we do what we do. So here is why I treat addiction:

Aside from the reward of restoring an individual's daily function, I enjoy the challenge of working with a condition extending far beyond the typical reversible organic disruption we see with the traditional medical conditions--one involving psychological, social and biological components interacting independently or in concert. While reversing the brain changes that occur in addiction through medications is vital to my practice, individuals also require assistance in developing skills to cope with unavoidable negative and stressful life experiences as well as how to experience pleasure

3

and gain meaning out of their every day's life without the use of a substance. Coming off substances carries numerous implications for an individual. It leaves them with underlying mental health conditions masked by substance use, with the guilt and shame of behaviors while under the influence, with legal and financial consequences, and lack of support due to broken relationships. This leaves the individual highly vulnerable to return to use. The disease itself represents the underlying neurophysiological (brain) changes, yet the social and psychological components driving and maintaining the disease require an interdisciplinary, team approach. To this end, I require help from psychologists, counselors, social workers and case managers, law enforcement, the patients' families and other medical specialties.

Before training in addictive disorders, I regarded individuals actively suffering from addictions as manipulative, dishonest and deceiving. I heard stories of patients lying about symptoms to obtain medications with abuse potential, stealing prescription pads and forging physicians' signatures, "doctor shopping" or visiting multiple physicians for abusable prescriptions. Treating medical and psychiatric conditions was a nightmare as such individuals were often nonadherant to treatment and rarely focused achieving goals. Through working with them in various settings I began to understand the nature of the disease and started seeing them in a different light. Following a patient from initial detoxification to

4

progression through residential programs, brings out some striking differences. Over the course of 28 days, I am able to see that these are not the same people we see when substance has control of their lives. When in active use, their values, motivation, decision making and judgement processes are masked by the substance and it is the substance driving them towards a particular pattern of functioning. During active addiction their mind is completely preoccupied with doing everything required to obtain the substance and the substance is at the center of everything they do. Family and work do not matter, committing crime to obtain the substance (or means to procure the substance) is acceptable however contrary to their values, and giving up a life-time of work to use is seen as an acceptable cost. This lying, manipulative person with criminal tendencies is not the same when clean. When in recovery, this individual is capable of successfully weighing the risks and benefits of their actions, they have moral values, they love their family, and they regain goals and aspirations.

The cumulative effects of the disease not only kills the individual, but also places an extreme burden on the healthcare providers, society, and, most notably, their families. From a medical standpoint it is impossible to manage hypertension when someone has a cocaine use disorder. It too would be difficult for someone with an alcohol problem to adhere to a thrice daily insulin regimen. Drug overdoses are now the number one silent killer in America and substance use has both directly and indirectly led to our recent decline in life expectancy.

With the recent declaration of the opioid crisis as a "national emergency," we all need to take steps to prioritize the treatment of addiction. We can all make a difference, whether that is a family member gaining a better understanding of how to support a loved one and get them treatment, or the legal system transitioning from a punitive stance to a treatment oriented approach, or medical providers modifying their approach to better engage patients in substance use treatment. We all need to make some changes.

INTRODUCTION

"Why can't he just stop?"

"She chose to keep using..."

"He will have to pick between us or the drug"

"He stole to support his habit, so jail is what he deserves"

These are common themes that have emerged during my interactions with patients' families and loved ones. Even to this day, society tends to view addiction as a moral failure. The individual is assumed to have capacity to decide whether they use or not. Additionally, they are generally held accountable for the consequences of their actions while actively using. Often there is an expectation that once an individual is through detoxification, they are to function like the average individual without medications given the common belief that "one is not sober if dependent on a drug." This is the current state of how society views addiction. Throughout this book I will attempt to shine light on the neurobiological processes occurring in addictive disorders in an attempt to provide some insight and to better understand the individual's experience. I will also discuss the role of family and social support in the life of someone battling an addiction and how they can best help the individual.

Before I begin, it is important to take a look at the current landscape of addiction in the United States. In the past year, close to 10% of Americans over 18 years of age were diagnosed with having a substance use disorder. In the same year, close to half of all 12th grade students endorsed experimenting with illicit drugs and 6% admitted to daily marijuana use. Adolescents are also staring early, with the average age of first time marijuana use being 12 years of age—a time when the brain is still growing and developing. For several years now, drug overdoses remain the leading cause of death in Americans under the age of 50. In 2017, a total of 72,000 Americans died by overdose—representing a 10% increase over the prior year. In addition to a growing number using opioids, there is concern that novel synthetic opiates such as Fentanyl are both much more potent and cheaper.

While the mortality associated with overdose has been fairly visible publically, some substances are more insidious in nature and tend to increase morbidity by a slower, more gradual, demise. Tobacco, for example, is the leading cause of preventable death and disease world-wide---smokers live on average 10 years less than non-smokers. Smoking related illnesses include cancers, heart disease, respiratory disease, autoimmune conditions among others. Recent surveys indicate that 7 out of 10 smokers want to stop and that of these more than half have made an unsuccessful attempt in the last year. Without prescription medication to aid in cessation the odds of success are greatly against the individual.

Substance abuse does not simply lead to health problems, disability, and death, but also causes significant emotional pain to the individual, their families, and community. Through my work with individuals with addictions, I have heard horrendous stories of the lengths to which patients have gone to procure substances, the shameful behaviors indulged while intoxicated, and the harrowing experience of withdrawal. Individuals with addictions often fail to meet responsibilities at work, school or home—resulting in job loss, alienation from family, discord with loved ones, and a decline in socioeconomic status. Individuals are also predisposed to criminal behaviors and approximately half of individuals with addictions reside in jails. Strikingly, the same individual when clean, reflecting on his past, could earnestly state, "that was not me, I don't know why I would do such a thing—it goes against all my values". This resultant feeling of guilt and shame in combination with a lack of social support (damaged relationships), very often prompts the individual to return to use and drives a never-ending cycle.

An important concept to consider is that not everyone who uses a substance has an addiction to that particular substance. We are all familiar with the social norm of having the occasional drink after work or in celebration. Typically, under such circumstances, individuals are not intoxicated, are able to return home, carry on with their regular activities, and arise the next day for work without the need or thought about a drink until the next socially appropriate context. There too, are those individuals prescribed pain pills after a surgery or acute injury that take their medication as prescribed—by mouth and not through any other route, at the intervals recommended as needed to manage pain. Once healed, they stop use, leave the remaining pills in the cabinet and are able to return to their normal life without a second thought. Recreational use of a substance and addiction to the same substance are very different, although they lie on a spectrum with a complex set of correlations that will be discussed later.

To provide the reader with context for the physician's perspective, we shall turn our attention to diagnosis and the criteria and symptoms set forth by the American Psychiatric Association. The Diagnostic and Statistical Manual of Mental Disorders (DSM), fifth Edition, or simply the DSM 5, represents the gold standard for psychiatric diagnosis and is based on decades of research and clinical knowledge. Ten separate classes of drugs are defined with some classes remaining loosely defined to accommodate emerging agents. For a diagnosis of an addictive disorder (a substance "use disorder"), at least two of 11 criteria must be met. The more that are checked off the higher the severity of the addiction. So what are the 11? Let's have a look, and we can further categorize these 11 into 4 main categories:

Category 1: Risky use of a substance, such as drinking when driving, or drinking despite having liver disease:
1. Recurrent use in physically hazardous situation
2. Continuing use despite negative physical and psychological consequences

Category 2: Physical dependence on a substance:
3. Tolerance to the effect of the substance requiring higher and higher amounts to produce the desired effects*
4. Withdrawal symptoms emerging when abruptly stopping use which can be relieved by resuming substance use*

    *Of note, special considerations are made for individuals who are prescribed medications such as popular anti-anxiety medications "Xanax" or "Ativan" which, if taken long term, will lead to development of tolerance and eventually withdrawal in the majority of patients taking the medications according to instructions.

Category 3: Impaired or loss of control over use of the substance:

5. Using the substance in larger amounts, or over longer periods of time, than it was intended to by the individual

6. Persistent desire to cut down on use of the substance or multiple unsuccessful attempts at cutting down or stopping use altogether

7. Spending a great deal of time obtaining the substance, using it, or recovering from its effects.

8. Cravings or intense desire to use

Category 4: Social impairment caused or exacerbated by use of the substance:

9. Failure to fulfill obligations at work, home or school due to substance use

10. Interpersonal problems and deteriorating relationships caused by or exacerbated by use of the substance

11. Important social, occupational or recreational activities given up or reduced due to use of the substance

During our diagnostic interview with the patient and family we listen for, and ask questions to determine how an individual's history and current presentation might fulfil these 11 criteria.

THE DISEASE

Physicians are afforded the guidance of the previously discussed 11 criteria in making the diagnosis of a substance use disorder. As for family members, I cannot fully appreciate the pain, suffering, and frustration experienced when a loved one breaks the promise to stop using, lies or steals to support his use, or even causes physical and psychological harm while under the influence. What about the individual with the active addiction? What does he feel during the midst of the disease? To appreciate the addict's experience, I utilize an exercise that involves holding one's breath. Here, we will imagine air to be our substance of choice and attempt not to use it. We will try our best to not take a breath—this will initially seem fairly easy. Add the incentive of $1,000,000 prize if we can hold our breath for 10 minutes. As time passes, we will start doubting ourselves. As it becomes uncomfortable, we will begin craving to take that breath and nothing else around us will matter, including the valued prize for 1 million dollars. Our body will signal that it needs us to take that breath and eventually our willpower and motivation to cash in on that lump sum of money will be meaningless. Unless we get oxygen in our lungs by some other means, we will succumb to taking that breath. With addiction, the brain is used to getting and requires the substance (oxygen in our analogy). Nothing else matters but the drug and it craves it in a very similar way to the way we crave oxygen in our exercise. There comes a time when nothing else but that matters.

There are four "C's" that categorize observable behaviors exhibited either alone or in combination by those suffering from this disease. First C represents control, rather the lack of control. Part of what distinguishes an individual with alcohol use disorder from her peers is his ability to control his drinking and stop after one or two beers. The second C represents compulsion, or the desire to persistently and repeatedly utilize the substance over and over again. In time this may not lead to the reward or euphoria as it once did. Continued use may simply relieve uncomfortable feelings of withdrawal. The third C represents continued use despite knowledge of the harm. Many of my patients can recite the entire list of medical conditions associated with ongoing substance use either directly or indirectly. Even those, such as physicians, with a deep understanding of the underlying physiological processes of disease progression will continue to consume and suffer consequences.. I have treated patients on parole for legal charges required to produce clean urine toxicology screens in order to avoid jail. Despite their understanding and appreciation that continued use would mean return to jail, they were unable to abstain from smoking marijuana. The fourth and last C stands for craving. Some may have dreams about using, some may find themselves day dreaming about procuring it, and there too are others, such as smokers, who can describe feelings of "almost tasting it" and wanting to have a cigarette so badly they feel like they are crawling out of their skin.

In the medical profession we study disease, learn about what exactly happens at a cellular level, and then develop treatments that target the identified processes. Take diabetes as an example— we know the disease results from either the body's inability to produce insulin (leading to impaired ability to absorb sugars) or the body's inability to utilize the insulin effective (which has the same outcome). When treating the condition, we therefore utilize external insulin in the former or agents that sensitize the body to insulin in the latter. We also educate the family of the diabetic on the condition and the steps required to successfully manage this lifelong condition. It is important that they understand that there will be episodes when blood sugars will be out of whack (e.g. infection) and therefore the diabetic may need short term hospitalization for stabilization. During this time the family should be trained to respond to the emergency and to support the individual. Fairly straight forward in the case of diabetes. However, when someone suffers from an addiction, our society tends to blame the individual, perhaps incarcerate him where he or she has no access to treatment. His family may break ties with him and overall relapses are viewed as complete failures. It would be highly peculiar if diabetes was handled in a similar manner. This discrepancy, must in part be attributed to the fact that what we cannot see and quantify is difficult to understand. Does addiction have any physiological basis akin to diabetes? Are the 4 Cs perhaps something we can measure in the same way blood sugar is for diabetes? In recent years, exciting new developments such as enhanced brain imaging, gene targeting and pharmacological options have made it possible to better conceptualize addiction as a medical disease. Much too has been gleaned from animal models. Let's take a closer look!

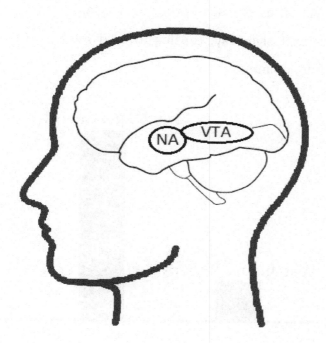

A particular structure in our brains called the nucleus accumbens (marked as "NA" on the diagram) is the focal point in addictions and it has aptly been termed the "pleasure and reward center". The nucleus accumbens is to addiction what the pancreas is to diabetes. The NA is connected in a circuit to another structure called the ventral tegmental area (or "VTA" on the diagram). Naturally rewarding activities such as sports, enjoying intimacy or a delicious slice of pie, releases a neurotransmitter molecule called dopamine (think of it as the equivalent of insulin's role in diabetes) from the VTA, which then travels to and activates the NA. This results in euphoria and reward. Brain imaging has demonstrated that this circuit is very active during the aforementioned pleasurable activities. All drugs of abuse produce the same effect, only in a much more explosive way, causing a rapid release of very large amounts of dopamine.

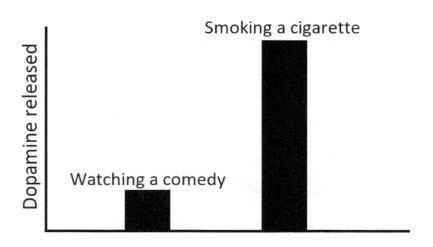

The circuit does not stop here, and other structures are involved. For example, the amygdala and hippocampus--structures typically involved in memory of emotions (especially fear) and the consolidation of information from short term to long term memory, respectively. If someone happens to enjoy a slice of pie when they visit grandma, the memory and association get stored away. In the future, when they see grandma, they will activate the memory center and cause a craving and desire to have a slice of pie. The hippocampus and amygdala are activated and the connection with the VTA-NA circuit is strengthened. The same thing occurs when patients suffer from cocaine addiction and crave the drug every time they pass a crack house. Yes, both pie and cocaine activate the same circuit. The "cue", whether it is grandma or the crack house, activates the reward circuit and triggers anticipation.

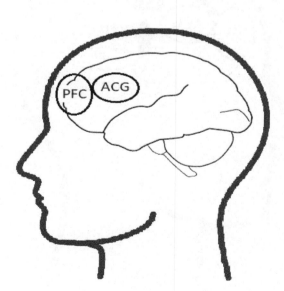

There are two additional structures that are very relevant to the discussion—the pre-frontal cortex (marked as "PFC") and anterior cingulate gyrus (marked as "ACG"). These regulate the overall motivational salience (relevance) and determine the intensity of the behavioral response. The PFC is important in managing complex processes such as reasoning, logic, problem solving and planning. Essentially, this is the self-control structure that prevents humans from pursuing urges or cravings all the time and motivates them to make rational choices and defer pleasurable activities. If you think of the VTA-NA circuit activation as being the gas pedal of a car (the "Go!"), you can think of the PFC circuit as the brakes (the "Stop!").

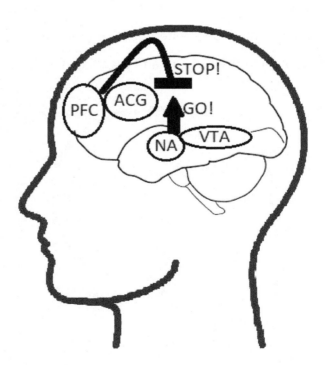

Drug use will activate the VTA-NA Go! circuit and the individual will experience euphoria. Initially the individual will have a sufficiently strong PFC Stop! circuit to exert control and regulate use. With repeated drug use, all the pathways we have discussed undergo "neuroplastic changes", a fancy term to describe how these pathways undergo strengthening and develop different connectivity among each other. The drug-induced burst of dopamine (much greater than that from natural rewards such as running, eating, etc), in the Go! circuits induces changes in cell signaling and in dopamine receptor distribution and sensitivity. This may result in weakening of the Stop! circuit connection and/or strengthening of the Go! pathway. The VTA can now release Dopamine in response to motivationally relevant events and the phenomena of learning takes place. The Stop! circuit signal weakens and therefore the ability to control and make choices is lost. With time and with repeated drug use, the individual will eventually lose the brakes and the Stop! circuit will not be able to overcome the much stronger Go! circuit, resulting in full blown addiction (overwhelming desire to obtain the drug, diminished ability to control drug seeking, and reduced pleasure from the typical biological rewards).

These are changes are responsible for the 4 Cs we observe in active addiction. Functional MRI brain studies (imaging) have demonstrated that in time, with sobriety and the development of coping skills through therapy, these changes revert and peak around 1 year. There are, still, lifelong changes in cell signaling and protein gene expression which converts vulnerability to relapse from temporary and reversible into permanent features of addiction.

We can see why it is difficult for someone to control addiction on their own when such changes occurred in their brains. In coming off substances, such as after a short detoxification, even though the individual no longer has substances in their systems, the brain remains geared to have a weak Stop! and a strong Go!. This makes the individual highly vulnerability to relapse due to craving the substance and seeking out the higher dopamine levels in their brain triggered by active use. With the assistance of relapse prevention medications, such a dopamine requirement may be satisfied by decreasing the Go! signal while behavioral therapy works on strengthening the frontal lobe's Stop! signal and also helps develop strategies for long term abstinence and for dealing with cravings and cue-induced triggers.

One important caveat here is that in adolescents, the brain development occurs in such a manner that the Go! signal is naturally stronger than the Stop! signal, even in the absence of drug use (hence the reason children tend to act impulsively and without good judgement). Adding substances to the picture only makes it more difficult for them to contain impulses, and they make exceedingly bad decisions when using. The frontal lobe, with the Stop! Circuits, is the last lobe to fully develop—with full development achieved around age 21. With the structural and connectivity changes induced by the addiction process, using substances at young ages can result in permanently stunted neurodevelopment, and in the case of marijuana, decreased intellectual abilities.

POTENTIAL CAUSES

Two genetically identical twin children adopted by different families produce one addicted to heroin and one teetotaler. How is it that a family adopts two children of different mothers, raises them in the same environment the same way yet one becomes an addicted to cocaine while the other does not? How is it that two co-workers under identical occupational stress can result in one developing an alcohol addiction while the other does not? Or, take for instance, the case of two patients prescribed pain medications with only one becoming addicted and the other seeing a full recovery? These are real scenarios I have encountered and speak to addiction's accurate and nuanced definition as "a chronic neurobiological disease with genetic, psychosocial, and environmental factors influencing its development and manifestations as well as recovery".

We are all equipped with a unique genetic makeup by the DNA that is inside each of the cells in our body. This determines our gender, the color of our skin, whether we can eat gluten and which qualities we possess. Some diseases are guaranteed at the time of birth (or conception for that matter). Huntington disease is one such condition. There too are conditions such as high blood pressure (hypertension) which has a moderately high 25-50% risk of inheritance. Studies have found that up to 60% of addiction vulnerability can be attributed to genetics. In my experience, most patients have parent or grandparent (or both) with addiction. Using genetic techniques, several genes driving opioid use and the development of an opioid addiction have been identified. Different versions of the gene can result in protection from, or risk for, dependence. Much is ultimately dependent on which version of a gene you inherit. Likewise, additional genetic factors, such as the version enzyme that process drugs, are encoded in our DNA. The enzymes involved in alcohol metabolism have been extensively studied. Of note, individuals of Asian descent tend to experience facial flushing when drinking alcohol and tend to have lower tolerance, resulting in earlier intoxication. These individuals tend not to enjoy alcohol. The manner in which alcohol is metabolized by the body is a two-step process: alcohol is metabolized to acetaldehyde and then from acetaldehyde to acetate. This is typically a smooth process in the majority of people, with acetaldehyde being cleared from the body at an appropriate rate. However, if the rate is too slow, accumulation will lead to flushing, nausea, and vomiting. Asians tend to have an enzyme that rapidly executes the initial step but have a much slower enzyme for the second, leading to acetaldehyde accumulation and the associated symptoms. There is a lower risk of alcohol addiction among Asian populations and therefore this combination of enzymes has a protective effect.

In the same way genetics play an important role in the development of addiction, they play a role in treatment, adherence to treatment, and ultimately the likelihood of achieving remission or abstinence. Studies have shown that the genetic heritability of treatment adherence for chronic illnesses such as high blood pressure, diabetes and asthma is about 40%, a rate that approximates heritability of treatment adherence in addictive disorders. The relapse rates in addictive disorders are comparable to other chronic diseases and range approximate 50-70%. Despite these similarities, there are stark differences in the way society views non-compliance and relapse in addiction and chronic "medical" disease, particularly in the setting of medication non-compliance.

As previously highlighted, genetics is only part of the story. Environmental factors such as stress, peer substance abuse, the influence of popular culture, and access have a critical role in the development of addiction. Access is a particularly important risk factor and it places individuals at risk of increased volume and frequency of use and, in turn, to increased risk of carrying the diagnosis of addiction. Alcohol is the most abused substance due to accessibility due to its legal status. Genetic studies reveal that explore alone is not sufficient to cause addiction, which is corroborated by the example of addiction rates in the population of patients treated with opioid pain medication. Only 20% of such patients develop addiction to opioids. Mental health play a significant influence on substance use disorders, with over 30% of the population with psychiatric diagnoses using substances. Many in this group attempt to, often unsuccessfully, regulate anxiety and other mood states. Personality traits such as impulsivity and constant pleasure seeking also predispose an individual to addiction. There too, are other diagnoses such as Attention Deficit Hyperactivity Disorder (ADHD), which untreated, has been shown to lead to substance use in adolescence. These children struggle with focus, concentration and tend to be impulsive and novelty seeking leading to them resorting to substance use.

Can having either a genetic predisposition or an environmental exposure alone lead to addiction? Maybe, but this is unlikely. Usually there is a combination of factors – acquiring the genetic makeup from parents that makes the individual enjoy or find the high in some way useful, after being exposed to the substance in the right context or under environmental stress.

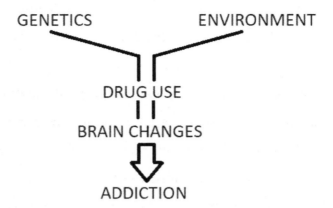

While genes can lead to greater than the average person's risk for addiction, they can also protect us from developing addiction—as seen in the earlier discussion of alcohol abuse in the Asian population.

Finally and often neglected, is the concept of priming the pump. Substances such as marijuana, that initially activate the Go! circuits described above, may increase the likelihood of developing addiction to other substances (e.g. heroin) that maintain activation of that same reward circuit. This has classically been coined the "gateway theory"—where consumption of culturally-perceived "harmless" substances eventually leads to "hard" drugs.

WHAT CAN ONE DO?

How can you, as a family member or friend, help a loved one battling addiction? This is a compressive chapter covering three important questions– how to help your loved one overcome the stigma associated with their disease, how to support them during active addiction and help them enter treatment and, finally, how to deal with a chronic disease associated with periods of relapse and remission (sobriety or abstinence).

Here are the main points, referenced within the chapter:

1. Learn about addiction and help fight the stigma.
2. Connect with peers like yourself.
3. Educate others and advocate!
4. Attend family sessions.
5. Encourage responsibility but do not point fingers.
6. Help but do not enable.
7. Use external pressure to motivate treatment.
8. Accept that relapses are common; use them as a learning opportunity and as a means to strengthen the relationship.
9. Recognize the importance of self-care.
10. Even with long-term remission, recovery should be a priority!

Stigma[1] associated with addiction is a significant challenge. Despite a great proportion of our society knowing someone with an addiction, few understand the biological processes underpinning the condition, and as a result, regard it as a moral failing on the part of the victim ("addict"). The legal system in the United States, relies heavily on punitive approaches to deal with the active substance use both initially and for relapses. Although the situation has seen gradual improvement, largely through education efforts, stigma and punishment remain commonplace. Stigma prevents an individual from reaching out for help, keeping them hidden in the active phase of their disease, and taking a mental toll and leading to frustration and continuous self-medication. Even in the case of sustained long-term recovery, issues relating to stigma can contribute to relapse, derailing years of progress. Particularly detrimental to the sufferer, is stigma from their family or support network. Individuals with addiction are often distanced from or by their families due to manifestation of the disease. Typically, the asthmatic suffering an asthma attack isn't abandoned by their family. The active phase of addiction, is a time when individuals are particularly vulnerable and require support. I hope that through the "The Disease" chapter of this book, I was able to help you develop a better understanding of the nature of the condition and the (very limited) control the sufferer actually has. One rather frustrating aspect of addiction is that the individual does not like using substances; they just are simply unable to stop themselves from using and doing everything possible to obtain and consume the substance. One approach to minimize stigma and build trust with the sufferer focuses on the choice of structure and vernacular used in conversations or discussions. A recent study found that terms such as "alcoholic" and "addict" carry more stigma than "person with substance use disorder". Allow me to illustrate an ideal conversational approach when talking about substance use, recovery, and issues related to addiction.

Don't Use:	Use:
"Substance abuser"; "Addict" "Alcoholic" "Heroin addict"	"Person who uses substances" "Person with a substance use disorder"
"Relapse" "Overdose"	"Recurrence of use" "Accidental drug poisoning"

It often important that family of patients with substance use disorders seek **support**[2] and surround themselves with others facing similar challenges. There are organizations such as Al-Anon or Nar-Anon which are geared at bringing together families of those with addictions, educating families, as well as providing support and access to additional resources. Another way to help reduce stigma is to **educate**[3] family members and friends that make up the sufferer's social and support network.   In recent years, many celebrities dealing with their own substance use issues have come out, raising public awareness and paving the way for non-celebrities to feel more supported when they are open about their battle with substances and seek help.

As mentioned earlier, our legal system has traditionally taken a punitive stance towards substance use which resulted in 60% of the incarcerated population serving time directly or indirectly for substance use. Some mental health courts are increasingly likely to drive individuals brought to their attention for substance related crimes towards addiction treatment with close follow up and monitoring rather than seeking imprisonment.

Before delving into the treatment process, let me discuss the issue of **relapses**[8], particularly given our earlier discussion of addiction's definition as "a chronic, relapsing and remitting condition". Treatment nonadherence and relapses are common amongst all chronic medical conditions. There is no cure for asthma, no cure for diabetes; but there are long term management options for both. Addiction is no different, and we have seen that brain anatomy and circuitry may be permanently altered to some degree and that there is no cure; however, there are long-term management options that allow for these changes to potentially be slowly reversed to some degree. Individuals with asthma and diabetes, like those with addiction, see relapse in the course of managing their disease. During a relapse, treat your loved one with compassion and understanding and facilitate or encourage them to seek re-entry into treatment as soon as possible. Use this as an opportunity for growth and learning from the experience, noting what contributed to the relapse and how this can be avoided and prevented. The goal of treatment is not to avoid relapses altogether but to decrease the frequency and duration of the relapses until they are few and far between and short-lived. Smoking cessation takes 5-6 attempts on average before a complete "quit". Learning from relapses and developing improved relapse prevention plans may eventually lead to permanent sobriety. Make your loved one feel supported and comfortable, so that when he or she relapses they can openly seek your help and support—getting back on track as soon as possible in order to avoid a full-blown relapse.

That being said, you do not want to make the individual feel overly comfortable with relapsing and developing an expectation of relapse and loss of self-efficacy and personal responsibility. **Accountability**[5] should be placed on the individual with the addictive disorder. External pressures such as consequences in relationships or employment are often the best drivers to someone changing and maintaining a behavior. Although punitive responses to relapse such as incarceration are extreme, having a parole officer, mandated treatment and requirement for negative drug screening can provide external pressure that leads to sustained changes in behavior. We have to learn how to best utilize the **external pressure**[7.1] since motivation to jumpstart recovery initially comes from outside (internal motivation is limited or absent as the brain has been high jacked by the disease process). Physicians do not differ from the general population when it comes to the development of addictions. It is estimated that, due to increased stress (the environmental component), they are at slightly higher risk for developing addiction than the general population. However, due to significant external pressures they are able to enter treatment programs and maintain sobriety at rates greater than the general population. Let us look at this more closely. Physician's external motivators such as the incentive to maintain a license and practice (considered by many a life calling) are highly contingent on achieving and maintaining sobriety. There are programs that monitor physician sobriety during their maintenance phase and work with licensing boards in order to identify triggers, imminent relapse, or early relapse so that they can intervene promptly and effectively.

During remission from substance use, family should remain supportive, express gratitude and acknowledge the importance of this accomplishment. Positive reinforcement provides the individual in recovery a sense of gratification and reward for their efforts and progress towards sobriety. One of the behavioral modalities for cannabis addiction is a technique called "contingency management" which is rooted in the concept of positive reinforcement. It works by having individuals check in with a counselor and provide urine samples to establish presence or absence of cannabis in their body. If negative, they receive a voucher to purchase goods. This positive reinforcement helps them attain a psychological reward and maintain the cannabis-free state (which got them the reward in the first place). Contingency management also provides a sense of accountability to the individual which can be empowering.

It is also important to encourage your loved one to always **put their recovery first**[10], even during remission. Recovery should be number one priority. Attending every Alcoholics Anonymous (AA) meeting and treatment appointment should be prioritized over any family event or work obligation. It is crucial that family members understand this point, and that they should not make the individual in recovery feel guilty for missing a birthday party or holiday get-together when in conflict with a recovery-related activity.

The "gold standard" for addiction treatment is the use of both medication to aid in relapse prevention (to weaken the Go! signal) and behavioral therapy (to strengthen the Stop! signal). Although there is evidence that, with time, the brain can return to its original state, there is limited data to suggest how long this process takes and to what extent the reversal takes place. Although behavioral approaches should be incorporated into daily life, there is insufficient data to suggest how long one should remain on abstinence promoting medications. Some experts advocate for a minimum of one year to 1.5 years for someone initially seeking help. After a relapse, it is advisable that the individual remain on medication for a longer period of time. However, no two people are the same, and treatment plans should be tailored to the individual's unique needs and strengths. Medications for recovery have a history of "taboo," as medications such as methadone for opioid use disorders do not conform to a model of total abstinence from psychoactive agents. Many will be familiar with the line "you are not sober if you are on methadone". Initially, twelve step groups such as AA were not welcoming to individuals on medications to help them abstain from using. However, with a much deeper understanding of the neurobiology involved in addictive disorders, the views on medication assisted treatment are evolving. We know that individuals stabilized on methadone function in society, hold down jobs and support their families. They avoid legal consequences from continued use and do no longer spend the majority of the day seeking out or using drugs.

"We change our behavior when the pain of staying the same becomes greater than the pain of changing"

-- *Dr. Henry Cloud and Dr. John Townsend*

Although a plethora of factors may lead an individual to seek treatment (legal mandate, medical concerns, familial conflict, financial or employment concerns), several studies have shown that **family pressure**[7.2] is the number-one factor driving individuals to seek treatment. I have, throughout my career, encountered many patients who presented seeking treatment in the context of marital discord, delivery of a newborn, or that parents will no longer provide financial support due to ongoing use. As previously mentioned, the brain is hijacked and therefore motivation initially has to come from the outside the individual in order to jumpstart the process. Family plays a vital role in early recovery. It is important to understand the **difference between helping and enabling**[6]. As family members, we do not want to assist the individual with addiction escape the consequences of their use. Providing shelter is generally considered helping, while providing money can often be enabling. Lying on their behalf or helping them conceal use from employers, spouses, and probation officers will only fuel the addictive process.

To further illustrate the importance of family support in early recovery, we will turn our attention to a type of intervention called Behavioral Couples Therapy. Here, the individual with a substance use disorder and their spouse sign a contract in which the two partners commit to maintaining sobriety daily, attend groups and to engage in a trust discussion where one partner discloses an intention to remain abstinent for the day and the sober partner offers support. The second part is engaging in relationship focused interventions, where positive feelings are shared and constructive communication is used to express feelings and discuss stressors. Aside from promoting sobriety, this intervention improves the relationship. This may seem silly at first, but evidence demonstrates that it works.

One previously highlighted aspect of addiction is the significant impact on the family. Aside from connecting with support groups, it is important to tend to your own mental health and emotional needs, and may involve individual therapy sessions. Practicing good self-care, exercising and staying on top of physical health are also crucial. You have to **take care of yourself**[9] first in order to best serve your loved one.

Let's take a step back. How do we, addiction psychiatrists, asses the interest one has in getting help? Individuals must be motivated for treatment and, as the quote above suggests-- when the pain of staying the same is greatest, that is when motivation is sufficient for change to happen. A model developed by Prochaska called the Stages of Change provides us with a framework to understand how motivated the individual is to get help. Starting at Stage 1, the individual is very ambivalent about even having an issue with substance use. This progresses to the individual identifying a discrepancy between their life goal and the (interfering) role substances play in achieving them. This in turn drives progression to subsequent phases and, eventually, the maintenance phase (and on occasion, relapse). Let's examine the Stages of Change more closely.

Stage 1 – Precontemplation:

Here, the individual is deep in their addiction, they do not think they have a problem, they are ambivalent, and cannot appreciate the impact substance use has on their life. Mechanistically, the Go! circuit has hijacked the Stop! decision-making and executive function circuit, and the brain is tricked into believing all is well.

Stage 2 – Contemplation:

The individual begins to realize that there may be an issue, however they are ambivalent about the need to seek out help. Often times, they will feel as if they can do it on their own. This is a window of opportunity to help them see the toll substance use has taken on their lives.

Stage 3 — Preparation:

The individual starts to make plans about how they might seek out help for managing their addiction.

Stage 4 – Action:

The individual has prepared mentally and enters treatment!

Stage 5 — Maintenance:

Long-term recovery with assistance from family, friends, peers and professionals.

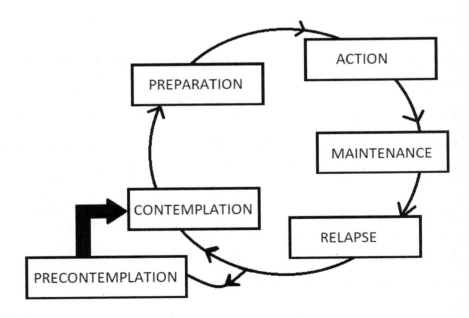

As addiction psychiatrists, we constantly evaluate which stage the individual has achieved and then attempt to move patients from one stage to the next using a technique called Motivational Interviewing. To be clear, motivation is not something we can provide the patient, but something we stir within them and attempt to strengthen. We subtly ask about the negative consequences of their use in order to create a mental list for them. Then, we juxtapose these consequences with the individual's goals and expectations for the future, gently allowing them to notice the discrepancy and inconsistency. Note that, motivation is dynamic and can fluctuate, taking the patient up and down the stages of change. An important goal in treatment is to rapidly recover from dips in motivation. Motivational enhancement can move one from a state of pre-contemplation to contemplation. You will have to learn not to confront the individual directly but rather roll with the resistances and defenses they might put up. This may be difficult at first, but confrontation and attempts to highlight negative aspects of ongoing use for them, will only push them away, create conflict, and the foster a feeling of not being supported. Behavioral change arises from the resolution of their ambivalence in a non-judgmental, non-confrontational, and non-adversarial manner. Engagement in twelve step programs and/or Cognitive Behavioral Therapy (CBT) can help the individual progress from the action stage to the maintenance stage. CBT is based the concept that learning plays a significant role in an individual's maladaptive behaviors. In practice, this means that patients are taught to identify and correct problematic behaviors (such as drinking to relieve stress) by applying skills that they learn in the therapy (e.g. identifying stress and using behavioral relaxation techniques as an alternative relief). It teaches one to anticipate problems that arise and engage their self-control through the development of coping strategies. It calls for self-monitoring emotional states, early detection of cravings, and identifying and avoiding risky situations that might promote use (e.g. avoiding parties where drugs are being used). Twelve Step programs are based on principles set forth by Alcoholics Anonymous in the 1930s. The model relies on psychosocial support provided in the group setting by other 'members' committed to sobriety. Individuals in early recovery are typically encouraged to attend 90 meetings in 90 days. One is also encouraged to find a sponsor (mentor) who has faced similar struggles with addiction, completed the program ("working the steps") and is now is able to effectively utilize the learned skills to maintain sobriety. Sponsors provide advice and guidance and are a critical point of contact (at any hour of day or night) when the "sponsoree" feels they are at risk for relapse. The individual commits to the twelve-step program of recovery, starting with step 1—acknowledging that they are powerless over the drug and that life has become unmanageable.

Let us conclude this section with an overview of the paths to recovery, including the different treatment settings, and the providers involved in the process. For the sake of example, we will take the case of an individual with alcohol use disorder with no past treatment. It is likely that abnormal tests at a primary care appointment, frequently missed appointments with a therapist, or visits with a psychiatrist will bring attention to the consequences of the individual's drinking. Perhaps open discussion and use of motivational enhancement strategies (often over time) help the individual overcome ambivalence about their use and motivate entry into treatment. They will in all likelihood require an initial inpatient hospital detoxification, as abrupt cessation can lead to seizures and death. This can typically last anywhere from 2-7 days. During detox, the patient is closely monitored by a physician and treated with medications to avoid seizures, stroke and hallucinations. Once the individual is detoxified, the most appropriate next step involves a stint at a rehabilitation center for 28 days (typical) to 90 days, focusing on the development of coping skills and strategy for sober living. A crucial aspect of this stage in the process involves therapy, with counselors and psychologists doing the majority of the work in conjunction with peer support and recovery peers. A physician will also follow the patient, adjusting medications, managing psychiatric and medical comorbidities, and following up on laboratory studies, etc. **Family**[4] often provides the important function of steady support and re-integration into their lives. Transition to the outpatient level of care can occur either directly or gradually through partial hospitalization or intensive outpatient programs. Such programs are structured such that the individuals spend time in counseling and groups during the day and return home at night. This often provides the individual with a more controlled return to daily life. Appropriate ongoing care involves regular physician follow up appointments and counseling sessions. Long-term strategy also involves attending peer support groups such as Alcoholics Anonymous and working with a sponsor. This provides the individual with accountability, which can be particularly valuable. Some individuals seek out additional accountability through regular urine testing, either through professional organization or private third-party testing.

Of note, individuals with chaotic and triggering home environments (e.g. spouse who drinks) or feel at particularly high risk for relapse, may be best suited in sober living—typically a community of recently sober individuals housed together for several months. Living in such an environment may be particularly desirable if the individual grew up around alcohol and lacked positive role models.

SOME CASES

I would like to illustrate a few fictional (yet realistic) cases that will help solidify some of the knowledge we have covered in the preceding chapters. Again, these are not real patients.

JOHN

John is a 50-year-old man who arrived at my office at the behest of his wife and daughter. A few days prior, he had called his wife at 1:30 AM, requesting that she pick him up from the local police station with bail money in hand. He had been arrested for his second DUI of the year. When initially confronted by law enforcement, John reported that he had only consumed a single beer and refused the field breathalyzer over sanitary concern. During our appointment, it also came to light he was fired from work last because his boss suspected he was intoxicated on the job. John was somewhat defensive in his recount and felt his firing was uncalled for and that the company was at a greater loss as he was their top earner. Subsequently, with his additional free time, he began spending more time socializing at the local bar with friends and consuming a "few beers" at home while watching TV. In the week prior to his presentation, John's wife filed for separation due to his behavior while intoxicated and continued drinking. Blood work indicated significantly elevated liver enzymes. The nurse noticed alcohol on his breath during blood work, which John attributed to having had the previous night. He could not provide an exact amount of alcohol he consumes, but states he does not drink "more than the average Joe". Curiously, he added that growing up his father drank significantly more than he currently did.

John stated that he wanted to get the visit over and done with, in order to satisfy his wife so that they could get back together.

A first look at John's case:

- *First let us examine factors that predispose John to developing addiction: genetic—his father likely had an alcohol use disorder hence some genetic predisposition, and context—increased stress and several unfortunate events that may lead to "self-medicating" negative emotional states with alcohol. Cultural factors are also in play, including his friends' preferred venue—the bar. The fact that John he feels compelled to use alcohol while watching TV points to an environmental trigger.*

- *As is so often the case, there is an external pressure bringing the patient to my office. He does not present because of his own desire to quit or recognition that his drinking is problematic. John's brain is misled by his activated Go! circuit, which leads to him to rationalize continue drinking in the face of negative consequences. He is truly blinded by his own brain when he thinks that he does not have a problem despite mounting evidence. At this stage, John is 100% driven by the activated GO! reward circuit and the Stop! prefrontal cortex is powerless by comparison.*

- *Fortunately, John's family is supportive, and they want to bring him to the attention of a medical specialist. Unfortunately, John is at the pre-contemplative stage and has little, if any, motivation to change. Motivational interviewing would be valuable in this situation.*

I start by asking John about what is important to him. He tells me that he wants to have a happy marriage, that he wants to see his daughter go to college, and that he would eventually like to get involved with the administrative branch of his company in order to curtail his involvement in physical labor. I inquire whether he feels that alcohol is any hindrance to accomplishing these goals. He responds, "Look, I can stop drinking if that is what you want," and proceeds to storm out of the room.

Noteworthy here:

- *My approach to John was non-confrontational and I did not attempt to point out the consequences for him, but rather, sought to have him identify the role alcohol plays in his ability to achieve his stated goals . I simply rolled with his resistance, attempting to have him develop discrepancy between his goals and the impact alcohol has on preventing him from reaching them.*

A week later, I see John in the waiting room on an early morning. He asks if I have a few minutes and informs me that after the visit his wife made him promise that he would not drink again, and was unable to keep his word. He noted that while he was able to abstain a few days after making the promise, and return to work after making amends with his boss, he found himself thinking, "I'll just have one cold one, it can't hurt." He ended up finishing the entire 12-pack he had purchased and attempted to hide this from his wife. . She, however, quickly detected the stench of alcohol on his breath. They ended up having a fight and she is again considering separation. Despite his efforts not to drink, John reported that he found himself in a similar situation—planning to consume a single beer and ultimately finished off the case. He recalls attempting to talk himself out of drinking, but then purchasing beer from the store later that same day. He is now questioning these bizarre phenomena.

What has happened:

- *The attempt at motivational enhancement was likely valuable in having John contemplate (doubt) his ability to control his drinking. He faces mounting external pressure from his wife and he is realizing that he does not have much control. He finds this both baffling and frustrating. He is entering the contemplation stage.*
- *John promised his wife he would stop drinking as a quick solution to her concern and a means to continue his drinking*

by denying the need for treatment. This is not the patient lying, but a symptom of the disease process. The patient truly believes that he can stop drinking and does not have a problem of control. Broken promises tend to destroy relationships and support systems, making it difficult for the patient to get the help they need and regain the trust of loved ones.

I inform John that I can assist him to achieve sobriety if he is so inclined. He states he is a strong man with a history of military service and that he can do this on his own. He feels that his recent attempts lacked sufficient motivation but has mustered up sufficient motivation to succeed this time around. He adds that he had a run of stressful days and felt that he required alcohol to relax.

What is going on now:

- *Excuses to relapse (such as having a few stressful days) are actually triggers for the patient but others may perceive them as excuses. Triggers can be either negative (getting fired from work) or positive (celebrating a birthday). These excuses are unconsciously created by the brain to enable ongoing use. Even with decades of sustained recovery, excuses can lead to relapse. I have often heard the case of older individuals returning to alcohol after 30 years of sobriety when their spouse passes.*

Three days later, John returns to clinic accompanied by his wife. He appears slightly intoxicated and tearful. He recalls having had several beers this morning before turning to his wife, with tears in his eyes, stating he "cannot control it". He reports that he will go to any lengths to stop drinking and seeks my advice. I help him enroll in a rehabilitation program where he spends 28 days. During this time he participates in individual counseling, group therapy, and programming geared at slowly involving his wife and incorporating her into his sobriety. John and his wife are able to strengthen their relationship through more open conversations, and set goals for life after discharge. He is started on Disulfiram (Antabuse) and agrees to have his wife administer this to him every morning in order to help him remain sober. He also makes plans to start attending local Alcoholics Anonymous meetings regularly and aims to complete 90 meetings in 90 days.

The take home:

- *During the active phase of addiction, the sufferer is blinded to an apparently obvious problem. Their reward circuits take over and brain prioritizes consumption of drug or alcohol above all else. Rational decision-making and values are diminished and have limited impact.*
- *At the right time, the right amount of external pressure coupled with behavioral techniques can help the individual*

see the discrepancy between their goals in life and the incongruous role alcohol plays in achieving these goals. Family is generally the strongest source of support and motivation to enter treatment and maintain sobriety.

- *Medication, behavioral intervention, and professional support are important components of a good treatment plan.*

MIKE

Mike is a middle-aged gentleman who has battled opioid use for the past five years. He was initially introduced to opiates when he was prescribed painkillers after a tooth extraction. In addition to managing his pain, he found that they relieved stress, allowed him to relax and provided him with sufficient energy to get through his busy day. When he completed his prescription, he turned to a street dealer. It was not long before he was offered the cheaper, and more potent, heroin. Shortly thereafter, he transitioned from snorting to shooting (intravenous). Mike has been through several cycles of detoxification, rehabilitation, and relapse. For the past 8 months, he has been on prescribed Suboxone (medication to assist in illicit opioid abstinence) and attending weekly outpatient groups and doing well in all aspects of his life. He has been facing increased work-related stress and was recently dumped by his girlfriend. To add insult to injury, his dog passed two weeks ago.

Not having a full grip on his emotions, he rather impulsively got in his car, drove to old dealer's neighborhood to obtain heroin, and finally used. Hours later, he was overcome by feelings of shame and guilt and thoughts that he was a failure. His distress fueled urges to obtain more heroin, but instead he decided to call his parents, who have been supportive in his recovery.

A first look at Mike's case:

- *The theory of self-medication describes individuals using substances in order to control their emotional states. For example, someone who feels anxious may be tempted to use alcohol or benzodiazepines to calm themselves. Someone who feels tired and lacks motivation may be tempted to use a stimulant like methamphetamine or cocaine. As an aside, over the long-term, these substances will eventually negatively impact mental states (someone who uses cocaine to help with apathetic mood will, in time, start to feel more depressed despite escalating use). Relapse triggers can also arise from negative emotional states as described above. It is important to learn to promptly identify these triggers and develop alternative coping strategies.*
- *Early identification of triggers and early action to address relapse are crucial determinants of prognosis. These can be*

taught through the Cognitive Behavioral Therapies described in the previous chapter. Confiding in family members and assuring that they adopt a nonjudgmental stance to relapse can facilitate seeking help early on and avoiding a full blown relapse.

Mike then moves in with his parents and enters an intensive outpatient program in addition to continuing his prescribed Suboxone. He is able to overcome the slip and continue the progress he has made. Mike and his parents become even closer. Mike learns from this experience, developing an additional relapse prevention contingency plan.

The take home:

- *Relapse is part of the disease process, it is not an indication that current treatment has failed. Addiction treatment requires lifelong commitment and priority. Lessons are learnt along the way. Use relapses as a learning experience!*
- *Reflecting back on this case, it is clear that the relapse y occurred long before Mike drove to get heroin. There had likely been changes in his mood, behavior and state of mind weeks prior. The accumulated stress acted as a trigger. Identifying those early changes could be crucial going forward.*

ANTHONY

Anthony is a young man in his early 30s who comes to my office because "I'm done using". He tells me getting suspended from work was a wake-up call for him and he wants to take the right steps towards recovery. He works in finance and two weeks ago his boss, a recovering person with alcohol use disorder, walked in on him smoking "crack" in his office. He was told to go home and not to come back until he gets help. The past few days he spent at home and realized he is unable to stay away from the drug which was a huge eye opener. He now feels tired all the time, spends the entire day napping and eating a lot. The cravings are getting very bad. He's been "meaning to cut down" for a long time but never realized it would be this hard. He tells me he should've realized he had a problem a long time ago as his girlfriend broke up with him last year over his use and parents no longer allow him at their house for family functions due to concerns that he might be bringing drugs in. He also has been falling behind on rent due to spending significant amount of money on obtaining the drug.

What is happening here:

- *Anthony accumulated a lot of reasons to realize he has a problem with substances and this helped him have the motivation to come in for help. His boss who is in recovery himself did not act as an enabler by covering up his use but rather provided just enough pressure for him to get help through the suspension until help is sought.*

- *Coming off a substance such as cocaine or any other stimulant will have a significant withdrawal manifested through fatigue, tiredness, oversleeping, overeating and low mood or dysphoria. Basically the opposite of its effects during use. Although these are not indefinite in duration they can promote the individual to resume use.*

- *Side note, going back to the self-medication theory discussed previously, this individual could've initially been using the cocaine to deal with these symptoms that he had prior, perhaps due to an underlying depression?*

I asked Anthony to tell me about how he started using. "Well, I was a pot head in high school, smoked weed every day, but that wasn't an issue. Then at a party while smoking I met some girls who said I should try cocaine. Instantly I was like 'wow' and haven't put it down since. I still smoke marijuana now but that's only when I get too high on coke".

What can we take away from this:

- *Remember the gateway theory we discussed in previous chapters? Our society views marijuana as being "harmless" and every year surveys show this is becoming more and more the case especially with more and more states adopting a recreational use stance. Not only does it activate the very same Go! circuit that all substances of abuse activate leading to development of addiction and potential for cross addiction (developing an additional addiction to another substance such as cocaine). Being a user also put Anthony in situations where he was around users of not just marijuana but other substances as well.*

- *Sometimes individuals alternate use of substances that have different properties such as here. Anthony uses marijuana now to calm down from the activated state the cocaine may put him in.*

I explained to Anthony the neurobiological aspect of addiction as described in "The Disease" chapter and the need to quit both substances at once rather than working on giving up one at a time. He was hesitant at first but later amenable. He tells me he is afraid he will relapse due to the symptoms he is experiencing now and having thoughts of how much better and more energetic he felt while using. I discussed with him potential admission to a rehabilitation center where he could be in a controlled setting while the symptoms pass and where he can begin developing skills to manage cravings and live life sober. He was very adamant that this is not an option but he would be willing to connect with a counselor and engage in an Intensive

Outpatient Program and try any medications I feel would be helpful.

What is going on now:

- *We have to work with the patient's preferences in order to empower them in their decisions and allow them to be in control of their treatment. Here Anthony wants to try the IOP where he can come to group therapy 3 days weekly and provide urine samples to ensure sobriety. If this fails, then I can discuss inpatient rehabilitation admission again with him (which would have been my ideal choice). The urine samples provide accountability to him, further assisting in his sobriety. We could even consider one of the Contingency Management approaches as previously described in this book where he can receive a voucher as positive reinforcement for every drug test that is negative.*
- *There are no FDA approved medications for stimulant use disorders. There are however some off-label medications with evidence for efficacy that may be able to assist with the low mood, low energy symptoms that interfere with his recovery.*

Anthony enters the IOP program and is able to develop the skills to maintain sobriety. He is able to return to work on a part time basis for now. He also reaches out to his parents and brings them in for some family counseling sessions with the therapist and this brings them closer together.

Closing remarks:

- *Family is an important component of an individual's recovery. Through family therapy, Anthony is able to strengthen the bond between him and his parents and make amends for all the wrongdoings in the past and the family is able to gain a much better understanding of what Anthony has been going though during active use.*
- *Recovery should always come first even if it means reducing the number of hours at work in order to attend IOP or do activities like meditation, counseling, etc that foster recovery.*

Made in United States
North Haven, CT
22 January 2022

15126791R00036